Reversing Heart Disease Cookbook

30 Plant-Powered Heartache to Heart Healthy Dinner Recipes

30 DAYS DINNER OPTIONS

NUEL VICTOR

Disclaimer:

The information contained in this book is for informational purposes only and should not be construed as medical or psychological advice.

The author assumes no responsibility for any actions taken or results obtained from the use of the information contained in this book.

Table of Contents

INTRODUCTION

Every year, millions of people across the globe deal with the devastating effects of heart disease, which impacts not only the sufferers but also their loved ones. Nevertheless, optimism persists. According to studies, switching to a plant-based diet may significantly improve cardiovascular health and even reverse the consequences of heart disease.

With an emphasis on plant-based foods, this cookbook presents 30 delicious and healthful supper ideas. Not only will these meals satisfy your hunger, but they will also fuel your body. We have taken great effort in crafting these recipes to ensure that they include heart-healthy, nutrient-rich foods with minimal saturated fats.

Whether you're currently following a plant-based diet or just trying to improve your eating habits, this cookbook has everything you need. To help you make nutritious meals that are full of taste, we've included nutritional information, advice, and thorough instructions with every dish.

Whether you're craving a substantial lentil stew or a delicious roasted veggie medley, you'll find a dish that suits your taste. Because we know it may be tough to make the switch to a plant-based diet, we've included some dishes that will make you feel good while still following the heart-healthy guidelines.

Keep in mind that this cookbook is only a resource to help you reverse heart disease, not a panacea. You may regain your heart health and embrace a full, vibrant life by making these plant-powered meals a regular part of your routine.

1. Mediterranean Farro Salad

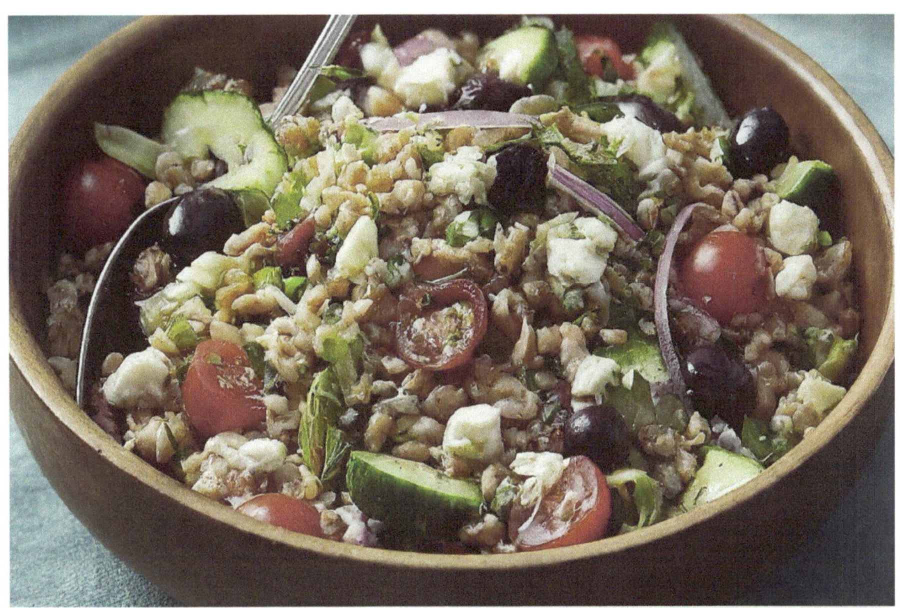

Ingredients

- 1 cup farro, rinsed
- 2 cups water or vegetable broth
- 1 cup cherry tomatoes, halved
- 1 cucumber, diced
- 1/2 red onion, finely chopped
- 1/3 cup pitted Kalamata olives, halved
- 1/4 cup fresh parsley, chopped
- 3 tablespoons olive oil
- 2 tablespoons lemon juice
- 1 garlic clove, minced
- Salt and pepper to taste

Prep Time:
1 hr 15 Minutes

Preparation

- Using a medium-sized pot, get water or vegetable broth to a boil. Add the farro, cover, decrease heat to low, and cook for minutes, or until soft and liquid absorbed.
- Cool the farro and mix it with the cherry tomatoes, cucumber, red onion, olives, parsley, and feta cheese (if using) in a big bowl.
- Mix the olive oil, lemon juice, minced garlic, salt, and pepper in a small bowl. After adding the dressing the salad, toss to mix.
- To enable the flavors to mingle, chill in the refrigerator for at least half an hour before serving.

Benefits:

Farro is a whole grain that's rich in fiber, protein, and antioxidants, making it great for the heart health as it reduces cholesterol levels and maintain blood sugar control. The olive oil and olives provide healthy fats that are beneficial for heart health, while the vegetables add essential vitamins, minerals, and fiber.

2. Quinoa Tabbouleh

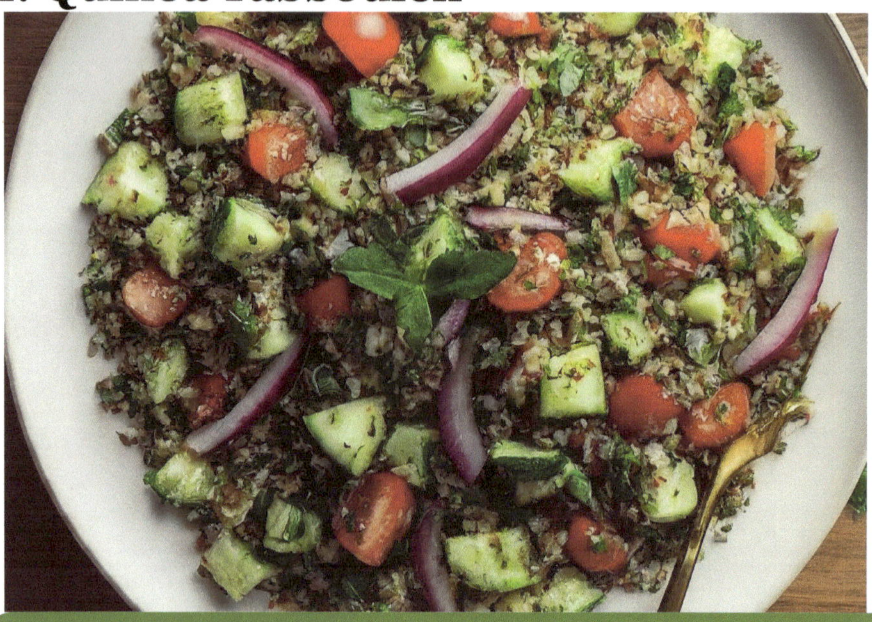

Ingredients

- 1 cup quinoa, rinsed
- 2 cups water
- 1 cup fresh parsley, finely chopped
- 1/2 cup fresh mint, finely chopped
- 2 medium tomatoes, diced
- 1 cucumber, diced
- 4 green onions, sliced
- 1/4 cup olive oil
- 1/4 cup lemon juice
- Salt and pepper to taste

**Prep Time:
1 Hr 35 Min.**

Preparation

- Add water to the quinoa in a saucepan. After bringing to a boil, lower heat, cover, and allow to cook for fifteen minutes, or until water is absorbed. Take off the heat and leave it covered for five minutes. Using a fork, fluff and let cool.
- Cool quinoa, green onions, cucumber, tomatoes, parsley, and mint should all be combined in a big bowl.
- Combine the following; olive oil, salt, lemon juice, and pepper in a small bowl. Drizzle the quinoa mixture over top and mix thoroughly.
- To enable flavors to meld, place in the refrigerator for at least an hour before serving.

Benefits:
Quinoa has all nine of the essential amino acids, which is a complete protein, which is rare for plant foods. It's also high in fiber and minerals like magnesium and iron, supporting heart health by lowering blood pressure and improving blood flow. The herbs and vegetables in this dish provide additional vitamins, antioxidants, and fiber.

3. Barley and Roasted Vegetable Pilaf

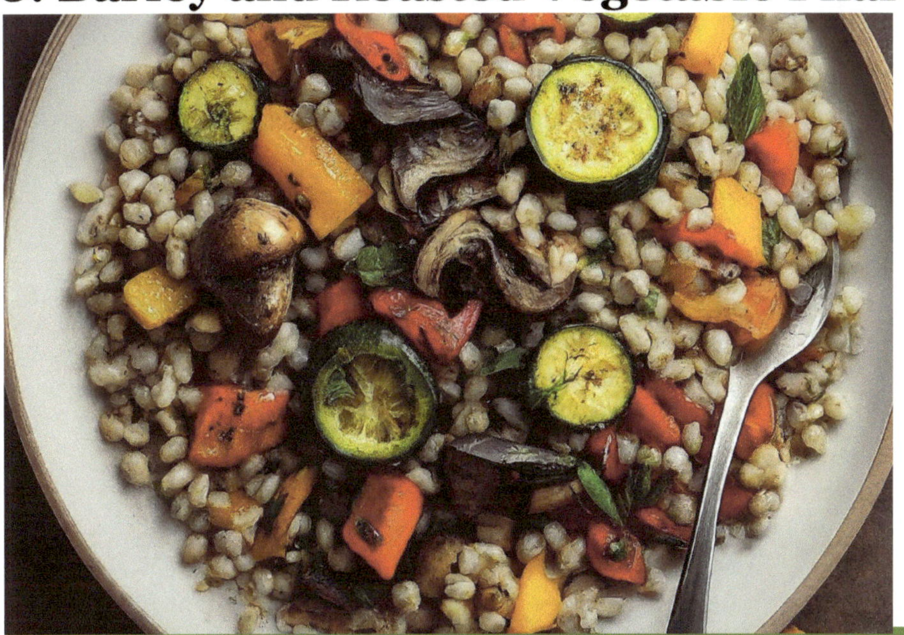

Ingredients

- 1 cup pearl barley, rinsed
- 2 1/2 cups vegetable broth
- 2 carrots, diced
- 1 zucchini, diced
- 1 red bell pepper, diced
- 1 onion, diced
- 2 tablespoons olive oil
- 1 teaspoon dried thyme
- Salt and pepper to taste
- 1/4 cup fresh parsley, chopped

**Prep Time:
1 Hr 5 Min**

Preparation

- Turn the oven on to 400°F, or 200°C. Combine olive oil, thyme, salt, and pepper with carrots, zucchini, bell peppers, and onions. Place on a baking sheet, then roast for 20 to 25 minutes, or until soft and starting to turn golden.
- While the veggies are roasting, heat the vegetable broth in a large saucepan until it boils.
- After adding the barley, lower the heat, cover, and cook for 45 minutes, or until the barley is soft and the broth is absorbed.
- In a large bowl, mix together cooked barley and roasted veggies. If needed, add more salt and pepper to the seasoning.
- Prior to serving, mix with some fresh parsley.

Benefits:
Packed with soluble fiber, barley is a heart-healthy grain that can help lower cholesterol and regulate blood sugar.

4. Wild Rice and Mushroom Stew

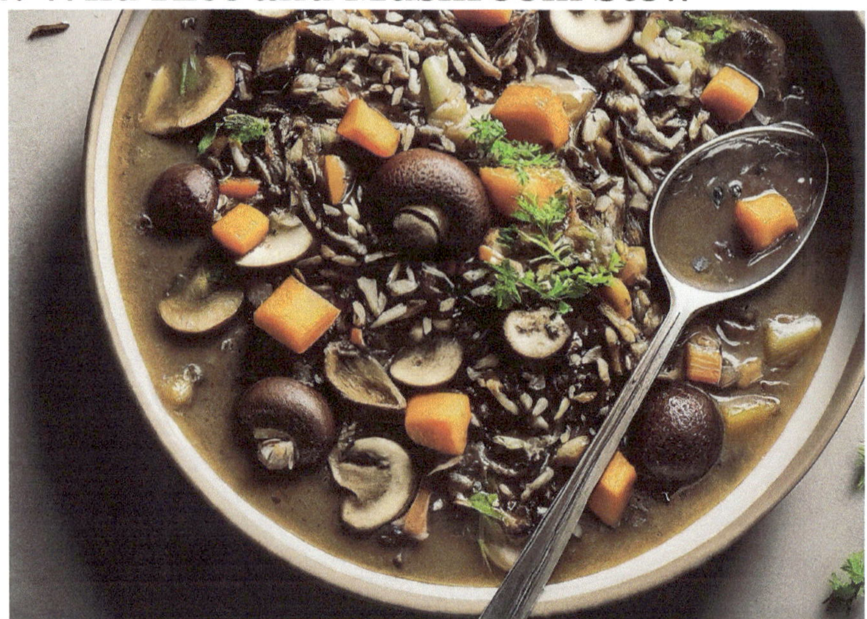

Ingredients

- 1 cup wild rice
- 4 cups vegetable broth
- 1 tablespoon olive oil
- 1 onion, diced
- 2 cloves garlic, minced
- 8 ounces mushrooms, sliced
- 2 carrots, diced
- 2 celery stalks, diced
- 1 teaspoon dried thyme
- 1 teaspoon dried rosemary
- Salt and pepper to taste
- Fresh parsley, chopped (for garnish)

**Prep Time:
Approx 60 Min.**

Preparation

1. Rinse the wild rice under cold water. In a big pot, heat the vegetable soup until it starts to boil. After you add the wild rice, lower the heat. Place a lid on top and cook for about 45 minutes, or until the rice is soft.
2. Lightly heat the olive oil in a different pan over medium-low heat. After you add the onion and garlic, cook them until they get soft.
3. Add the mushrooms, carrots, celery, thyme, and rosemary to the pan. Cook until the vegetables are tender.
4. Once the wild rice is cooked, add it to the pan with the vegetables. Stir well to combine.
5. Season with salt and pepper to taste.
6. Serve the stew hot, garnished with fresh parsley.

Benefits:
Fiber in wild rice lowers cholesterol and heart disease risk. The chemicals in mushrooms may lower cholesterol and inflammation, improving heart health. They are low in calories and fat. This stew's carrots and celery are high in antioxidants and fiber, which lower heart disease risk.

5. Buckwheat Noodles with Stir-Fried Veggies

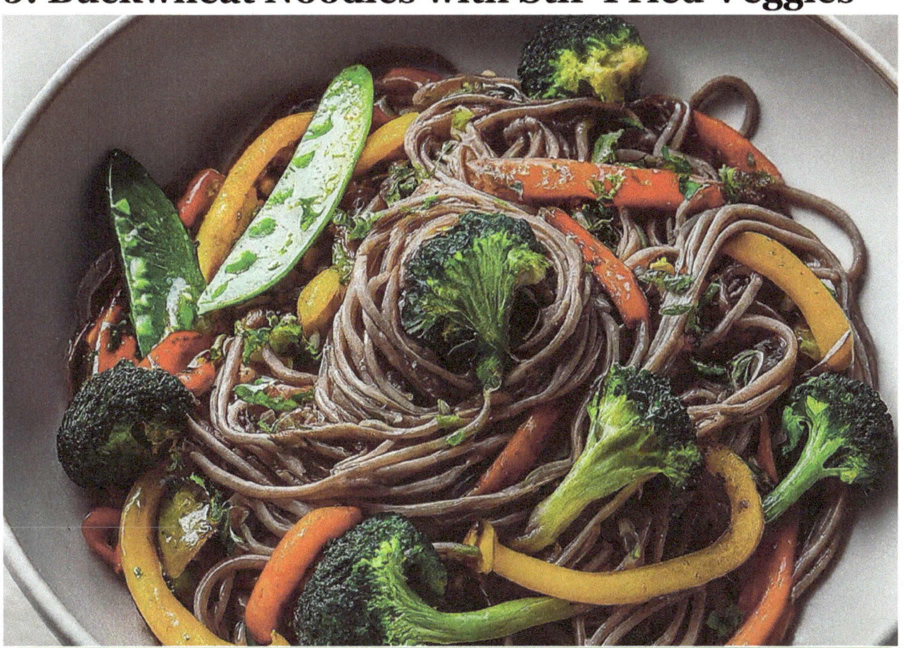

Ingredients

- 8 ounces buckwheat noodles
- 2 tablespoons vegetable oil
- 1 onion, sliced
- 2 cloves garlic, minced
- 1 bell pepper, sliced
- 1 zucchini, sliced
- 1 cup broccoli florets
- 1 cup snap peas
- 2 tablespoons soy sauce
- 1 tablespoon sesame oil
- Sesame seeds (for garnish)

Prep Time:

30 Minutes

Preparation

1. As directed on the box, cook the buckwheat noodles. Remove the water and set it aside.
2. Set the vegetable oil on medium-high heat in a large pan or wok.
3. Cook the garlic and onion until they are soft.
4. In a pan, add broccoli, snap peas, bell pepper, and zucchini. 5-7 minutes of stir-frying should get the veggies soft but still crisp.
5. In a small bowl, mix soy sauce and olive oil together. Add the sauce to the vegetables and mix it in.
6. Add the cooked buckwheat noodles to the pan and toss to combine.
7. Serve the noodles and vegetables hot, garnished with sesame seeds.

Benefits:

Buckwheat noodles are a good source of fiber and contain nutrients like manganese, copper, and magnesium, which can support heart health. The vegetables in this stir-fry, such as bell peppers, zucchini, and broccoli, are rich in antioxidantts and fiber, which can help lower the risk of heart disease. The use of vegetable oil and minimal added salt in this recipe can contribute to a heart-healthy diet.

6. Chickpea and Spinach Stuffed Sweet Potatoes

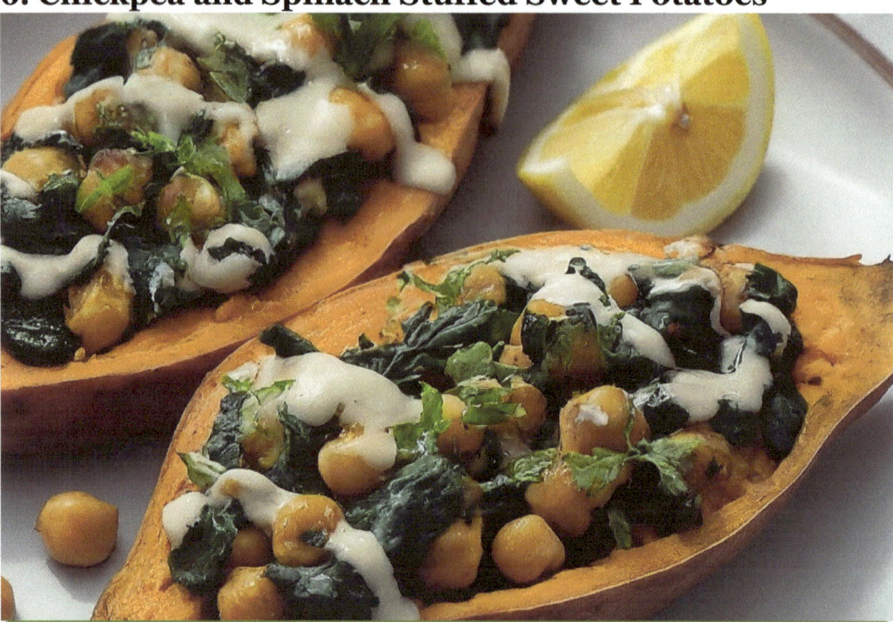

Ingredients

- 4 medium-sized sweet potatoes
- 1 tablespoon olive oil
- 1 onion, diced
- 2 cloves garlic, minced
- 1 can (15 ounces) drained and rinsed chickpeas
- 2 cups fresh spinach
- 1 teaspoon cumin
- 1 teaspoon paprika
- Salt and pepper to taste
- Fresh cilantro, chopped (for garnish)

Prep Time:

Approx 1 Hr

Preparation

1. Let's get the oven ready at 400°F (200°C).
2. Make sure to wash the sweet potatoes and gently prick them multiple times with a fork. Put them on a baking sheet and pop them in the oven for around 45-60 minutes, or until they become tender.
3. Heat the olive oil in a large pan over medium heat. Sauté the onion and garlic until they become soft.
4. Simply add the chickpeas, spinach, cumin, paprika, salt, and pepper to the pan. Continue cooking until the spinach has wilted and the flavors have melded together.
5. After the sweet potatoes are cooked, gently slice them open lengthwise and use a fork to fluff the soft flesh.
6. Spoon the chickpea and spinach mixture into the sweet potatoes.
7. Garnish with fresh cilantro and serve hot.

Benefits:

Sweet potatoes are packed with fiber, potassium, and antioxidants, which have been shown to have positive effects on blood pressure and heart health. Chickpeas are an excellent choice for those looking to incorporate more plant-based protein and fiber into their diet. They offer numerous health benefits, including the potential to lower cholesterol levels and promote heart health. Spinach is a fantastic leafy green vegetable packed with vitamins, minerals, and antioxidants that can potentially lower the risk of heart disease.

7. Lentil Taco Salad

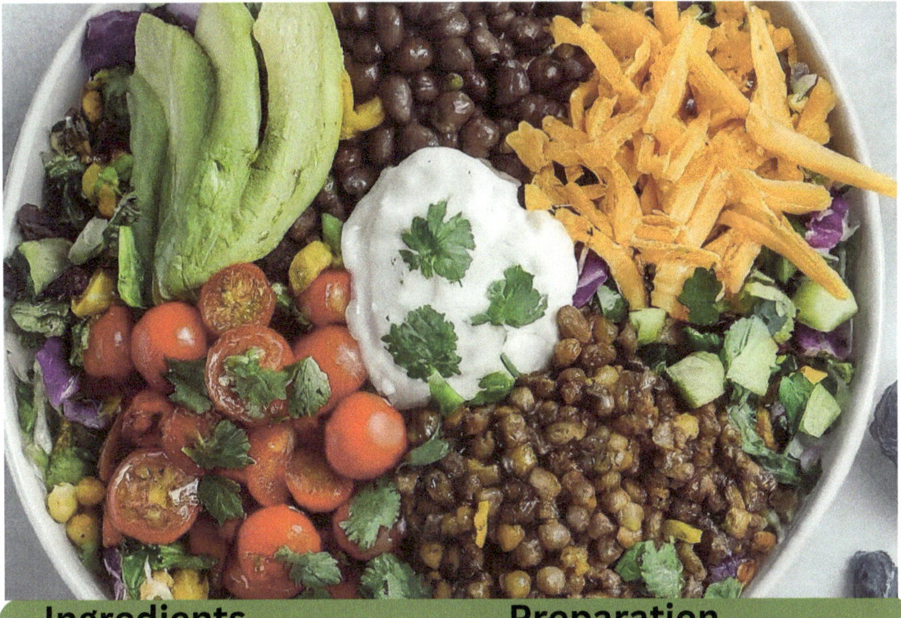

Ingredients

- 1 cup dried lentils
- 2 cups vegetable broth
- 1 tablespoon olive oil
- 1 onion, diced
- 2 cloves garlic, minced
- 1 bell pepper, diced
- 1 cup corn kernels
- 1 teaspoon chili powder
- 1 teaspoon cumin
- Salt and pepper to taste
- 4 cups mixed salad greens
- 1 avocado, sliced
- 1 tomato, diced
- Fresh cilantro, chopped (for garnish)
- Lime wedges (for serving)

Prep Time:
Approx 45 Minutes

Preparation

- Wash the lentils in cool water.
- Bring the vegetable broth to a simmer in a saucepan. Remember to add lentils and reduce the heat. Cover and simmer for 20–25 minutes to make the lentils tender. Remove any extra liquid and set it aside.
- Heat olive oil in a large pan over medium heat. Include onion, garlic, bell pepper, and corn. Cook the vegetables until they are nice and tender.
- Include cooked lentils, chili powder, cumin, salt, and pepper in the pan. Make sure to mix everything together really well and let it simmer for a few minutes.
- Mix the lentil mixture with the salad greens in a large bowl.
- Let's include some avocado, tomato, and cilantro in the salad!
- Don't forget to include some lime wedges to complement your taco salad!

Benefits:

Lentils are a great option for individuals who want to add more plant-based protein and fiber to their diet. They provide a wide range of health benefits, including lowering the risk of heart disease. The salad greens, avocado, and tomato are filled with essential vitamins, minerals, and antioxidants that are wonderful for promoting heart health. This recipe is perfect for maintaining a healthy heart, as it contains minimal amounts of saturated fat and cholesterol.

8. Black Bean and Corn Chili

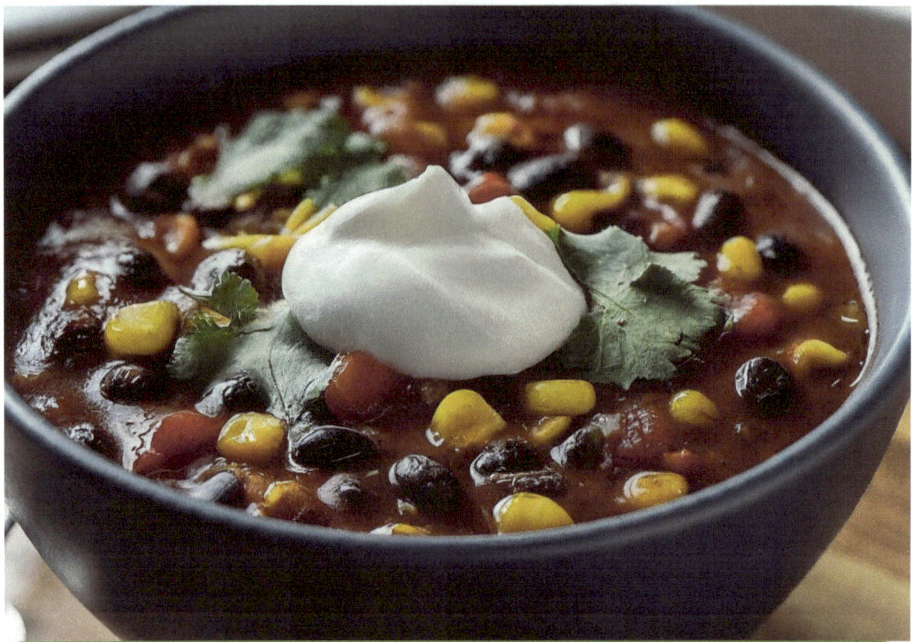

Ingredients

- 1 tablespoon olive oil
- 1 onion, diced
- 2 cloves garlic, minced
- 1 bell pepper, diced
- 1 jalapeño pepper, seeded and diced (optional)
- 1 can (15 ounces) rinsed and drained black beans,
- 1 can (15 ounces) diced tomatoes
- 1 cup corn kernels
- 2 teaspoons chili powder
- 1 teaspoon cumin
- Salt and pepper to taste
- Fresh cilantro, chopped (for garnish)
- Lime wedges (for serving)

Prep Time:
Approx 60 Min.

Preparation

- Heat the olive oil in a large pot over medium heat. Include the onion, garlic, bell pepper, and jalapeño (if desired). Cook until the vegetables are nice and tender.
- Let's go ahead and add the black beans, diced tomatoes, corn, chili powder, cumin, salt, and pepper to the pot. Make sure to stir thoroughly to combine everything.
- Bring the mixture to a gentle simmer and allow it to cook for approximately 30-40 minutes, giving it an occasional stir.
- Feel free to taste and make any adjustments to the seasoning if necessary.
- Enjoy the black bean and corn chili served piping hot, topped with a sprinkle of fresh cilantro and accompanied by zesty lime wedges.

Benefits:

Black beans are rich in fiber and protein, which can help lower cholesterol levels and support heart health. The combination of vegetables in this chili, such as onions, bell peppers, and tomatoes, provides antioxidants and nutrients that may help reduce the risk of heart disease. This recipe is low in saturated fat and cholesterol, making it a heart-healthy option.

9. Edamame and Avocado Spread on Whole Grain Toast

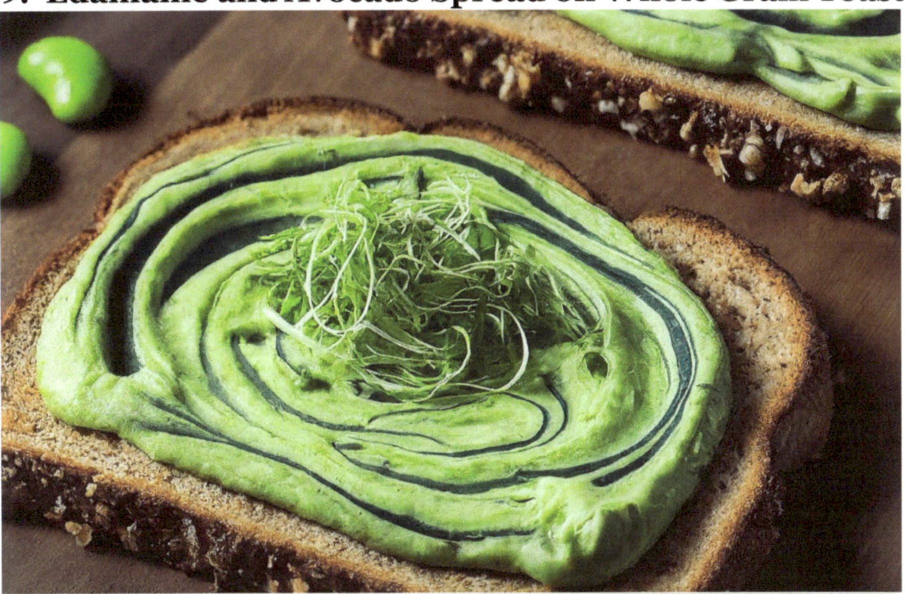

Ingredients

- 1 cup shelled edamame
- 1 ripe avocado
- 2 tablespoons lemon juice
- 1 clove garlic, minced
- Salt and pepper to taste
- Whole grain bread slices

Prep Time:

Approx 15 Min

Preparation

1. Bring a pot of water to a boil. Add the edamame and cook for about 5 minutes, or until tender. Drain and set aside.
2. In a food processor or blender, combine the cooked edamame, avocado, lemon juice, garlic, salt, and pepper. Process until smooth and well combined.
3. Toast the whole grain bread slices.
4. Spread the edamame and avocado mixture on the toast.
5. Serve the spread on whole grain toast as an open-faced sandwich or as a snack.

Benefits:

Edamame is a good source of plant-based protein and fiber, which can help lower cholesterol levels and support heart health. Avocado is rich in heart-healthy monounsaturated fats, fiber, and antioxidants, which may help reduce the risk of heart disease. Whole grain bread provides more fiber and nutrients compared to refined grains, making it a better choice for heart health.

12

10. Pea and Mint Soup

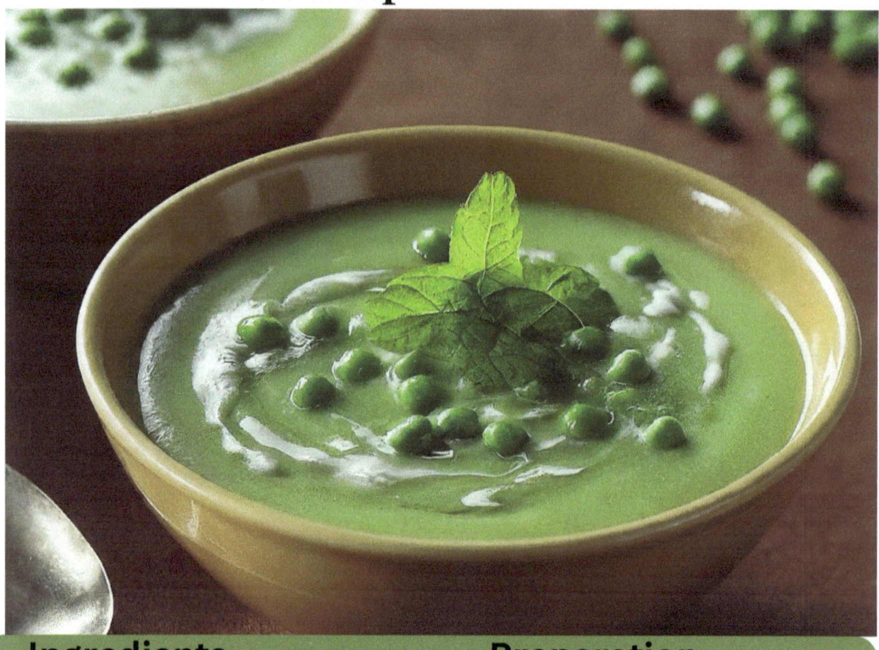

Ingredients

- 1 tablespoon olive oil
- 1 onion, diced
- 2 cloves garlic, minced
- 4 cups frozen peas
- 3 cups vegetable broth
- 1/2 cup fresh mint leaves
- Salt and pepper to taste
- Greek yogurt (for garnish)

Preparation

- Heat the olive oil over medium heat in a large pot. Sauté the onion and garlic until they become soft.
- Put the frozen peas and vegetable broth into the pot. Let it come to a boil and then lower the heat to a gentle simmer. Cook for approximately 10-15 minutes.
- Take the pot off the heat and gently incorporate the fresh mint leaves.
- Feel free to use an immersion blender or transfer the soup to a blender to puree until it becomes smooth.
- Season with salt and pepper to taste.
- Serve the pea and mint soup hot, garnished with a dollop of Greek yogurt.

Prep Time:

Approx 30 Minutes

Benefits:

Peas are a good source of fiber and contain heart-healthy nutrients like vitamins C and K, folate, and potassium. Mint leaves provide a refreshing flavor and may help aid digestion and reduce inflammation. This soup is low in fat and cholesterol, making it a heart-healthy option.

11. Roasted Cauliflower Steaks with Turmeric and Quinoa

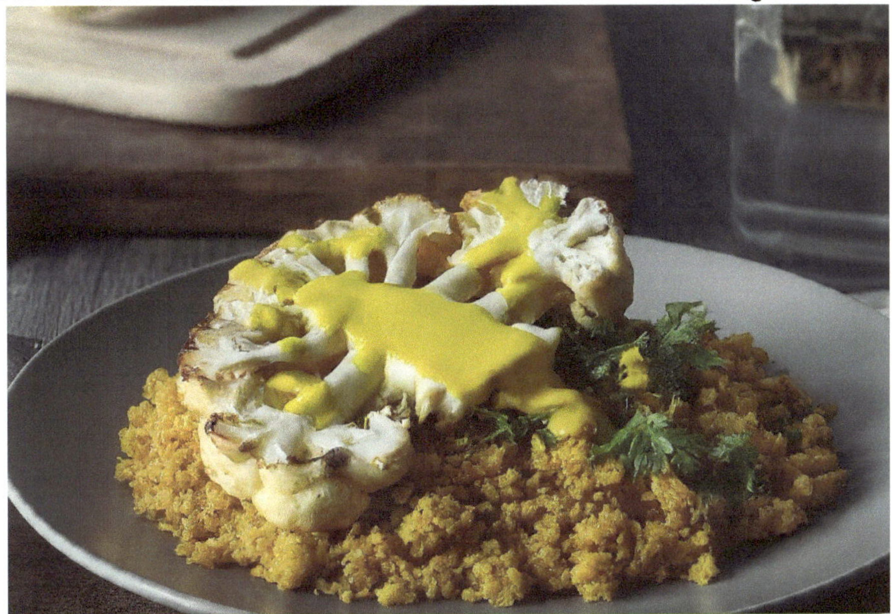

Ingredients

- 1 large head of cauliflower
- 2 tablespoons olive oil
- 1 teaspoon turmeric
- 1/2 teaspoon paprika
- Salt and pepper to taste
- 1 cup quinoa
- 2 cups vegetable broth
- Fresh parsley, chopped (for garnish)
- Lemon wedges (for serving)

Preparation

- Heat oven to 425°F (220°C).
- Remove cauliflower leaves and trim stem without removing head.
- Cut cauliflower steaks 1 inch thick.
- Mix olive oil, turmeric, paprika, salt, and pepper in a small bowl.
- Brush both sides of cauliflower steaks with turmeric mixture before baking on a sheet.
- Roast cauliflower for 25–30 minutes in a preheated oven until tender and golden brown.
- Quinoa should be rinsed with lukewarm water while cauliflower cooks.
- Boil vegetable broth in a pot, then add quinoa, lower heat to low, cover, and simmer for 15 minutes until cooked and liquid is absorbed.
- Fork-fluff the quinoa and season with salt and pepper.
- Over cooked quinoa, serve roasted cauliflower steaks.
- Serve with lemon wedges and fresh parsley.

Prep Time:

45 Minutes

Benefits:

Cauliflower is high in minerals, fiber, and vitamins. It may help minimize the risk of heart disease by decreasing cholesterol and maintaining normal blood pressure.. Turmeric includes curcumin, a substance with anti-inflammatory qualities that may benefit heart health. Quinoa is a complete grain packed in fiber and protein, which may help lower cholesterol and reduce the risk of heart disease.

14

12. Zucchini Noodles with Tomato and Basil Sauce

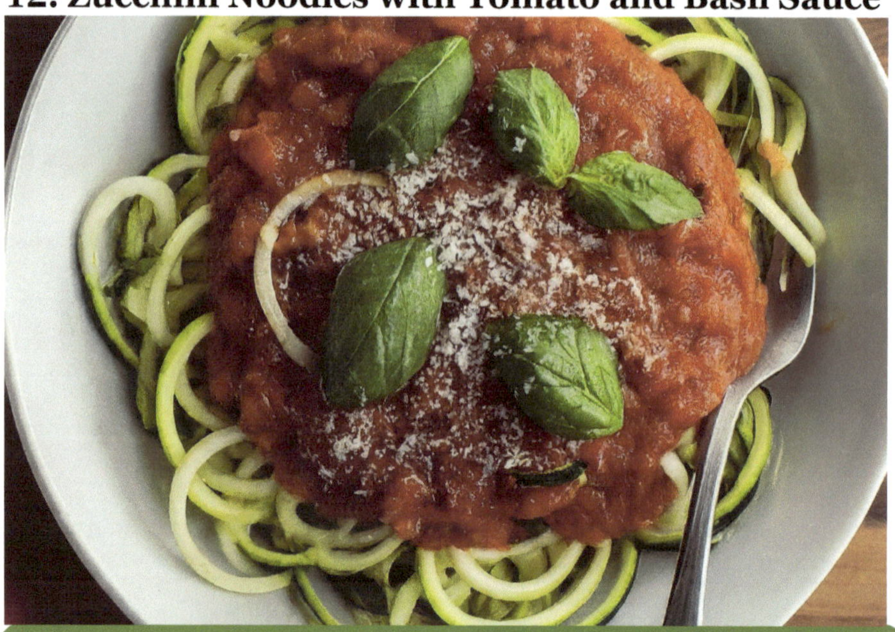

Ingredients

- 4 medium zucchini
- 2 tablespoons olive oil
- 3 cloves garlic, minced
- 1 can (14 ounces) diced tomatoes
- 1/4 cup tomato paste
- 1 teaspoon dried basil
- Salt and pepper to taste
- Fresh basil leaves, chopped (for garnish)
- Vegan Parmesan cheese (optional, for serving)

Prep Time:

15 Minutes

Preparation

1. Use a spiralizer or a vegetable peeler to create zucchini noodles from the zucchini. Set aside.
2. In a large pan, heat the olive oil on low to medium heat, then add the minced garlic and sauté until fragrant.
3. Add the diced tomatoes, tomato paste, dried basil, salt, and pepper to the pan. Stir well to combine.
4. Simmer the sauce for about 10-15 minutes, or until it thickens slightly.
5. In a separate pan, heat a small amount of olive oil over medium heat. Add the zucchini noodles and sauté for about 3-5 minutes, or until they are tender.
6. Divide the zucchini noodles among serving plates and top with the tomato and basil sauce.
7. Garnish with vegan Parmesan cheese and fresh basil leaves, if desired.

Benefits:

Zucchini is low in calories and high in fiber, which can help lower cholesterol levels and support heart health. Tomatoes are rich in lycopene, an antioxidant that may help reduce the risk of heart disease. Basil contains compounds that may help lower blood pressure and reduce inflammation, which can benefit heart health.

13. Stuffed Acorn Squash with Wild Rice Medley

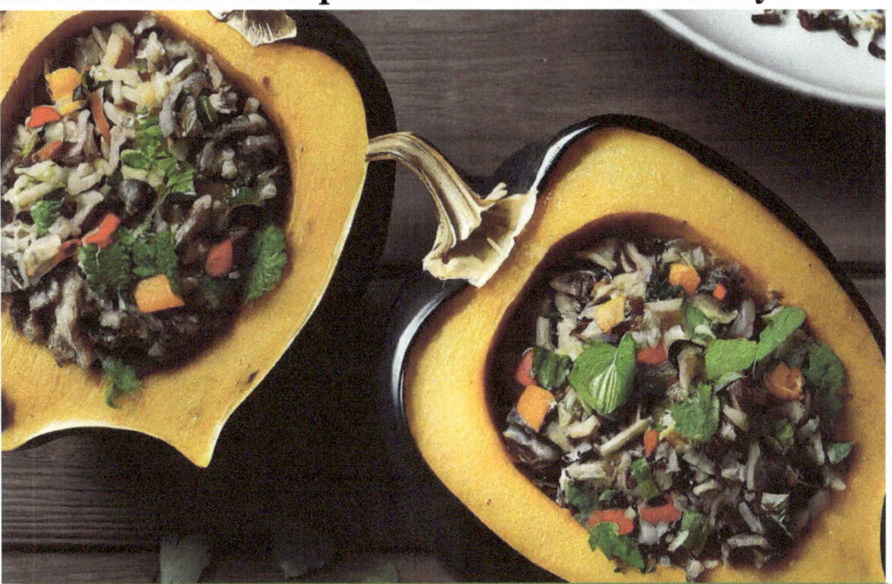

Ingredients

- 2 acorn squash
- 1 cup wild rice
- 2 cups vegetable broth
- 1 tablespoon olive oil
- 1 onion, diced
- 2 cloves garlic, minced
- 1 carrot, diced
- 1 celery stalk, diced
- 1/2 cup dried cranberries
- 1/2 cup chopped pecans
- 1 teaspoon dried thyme
- Salt and pepper to taste
- Fresh parsley, chopped (for garnish)

Prep Time:
1hr 15 Minutes

Preparation

1. Get the oven to 400°F (200°C).
2. Cut the acorn squash in half lengthwise and remove the seeds.
3. Bake the squash halves cut-side down on a baking pan for 30–40 minutes until soft.
4. While waiting, rinse wild rice in cold water.
5. Boil vegetable broth in a pot. Add the wild rice, lower the heat to low, cover, and simmer for 45–50 minutes until cooked and liquid is absorbed.
6. In a separate pan, heat olive oil on medium. Add onion, garlic, carrot, and celery. Sauté veggies until soft.
7. Add the cooked wild rice, dried cranberries, chopped pecans, dried thyme, salt, and pepper to the pan. Stir well to combine.
8. Once the acorn squash is cooked, fill each half with the wild rice medley.
9. Return the stuffed squash back to the oven and bake for an additional 10 minutes.
10. Serve the stuffed acorn squash hot, garnished with fresh parsley.

Benefits:

Acorn squash contains fiber, potassium, and antioxidants that decrease blood pressure and heart disease risk. Wild rice, a complete grain rich in fiber and minerals, may decrease cholesterol and improve heart health. Pecans are a heart-healthy nut that contains monounsaturated fats and antioxidants, which may help reduce the risk of heart disease.

16

14. Eggplant Rollatini with Spinach and Ricotta (Vegan)

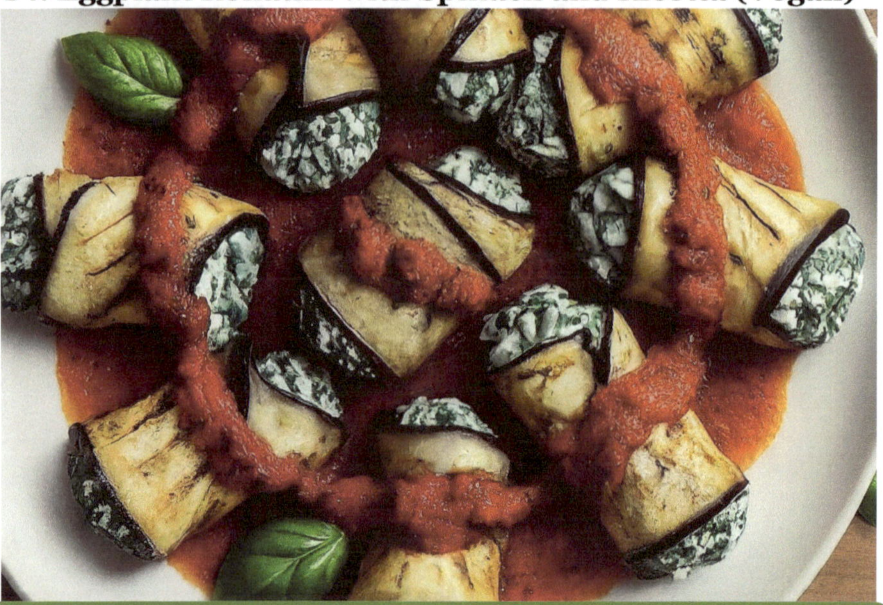

Ingredients

- 2 large eggplants
- 2 tablespoons olive oil
- 1 onion, diced
- 3 cloves garlic, minced
- 8 ounces fresh spinach
- 1 cup tofu ricotta (store-bought or homemade)
- 1/4 cup nutritional yeast
- 1/2 teaspoon dried oregano
- 1/2 teaspoon dried basil
- Salt and pepper to taste
- 2 cups marinara sauce
- Vegan mozzarella cheese (optional)
- Fresh basil leaves, chopped (for garnish)

Prep Time:

1 hr

Preparation

1. Preheat the oven to 375° Fahrenheit (190° Celsius).
2. Cut the eggplants lengthwise into 1/4-inch-thick slices.
3. Place the eggplant slices on a baking pan and brush with olive oil on both sides. Bake in a warm oven for 15-20 minutes, or until soft.
4. Meanwhile, warm a tiny quantity of olive oil in a pan over medium heat. Sauté the chopped onion and minced garlic until softened.
5. Cook the fresh spinach in the pan until wilted.
6. In a mixing dish, combine the tofu ricotta, nutritional yeast, dried oregano, dry basil, salt, and pepper. Mix thoroughly.
7. After the eggplant slices are cooked, take them from the oven and allow them to cool somewhat.
8. Spread a dollop of the tofu ricotta mixture on each eggplant slice. Top with a tablespoon of spinach mixture and fold up the slices.
9. Place the coiled eggplant slices in a baking dish and cover with marinara sauce.
10. Bake in the oven for 20-25 minutes, or until well heated.
11. If preferred, sprinkle vegan mozzarella cheese over the rollatini and bake for an additional 5 minutes, or until melted and bubbling.
12. Garnish with fresh basil and serve hot.

Benefits:

Eggplant is low in calories and high in fiber and antioxidants, which may help lower your chance of developing heart disease. Spinach is high in vitamins, minerals, and antioxidants, which promote heart health. Tofu ricotta is a plant-based alternative to traditional ricotta cheese, and it is lower in saturated fat and cholesterol

17

15. Sweet Potato and Black Bean Enchiladas

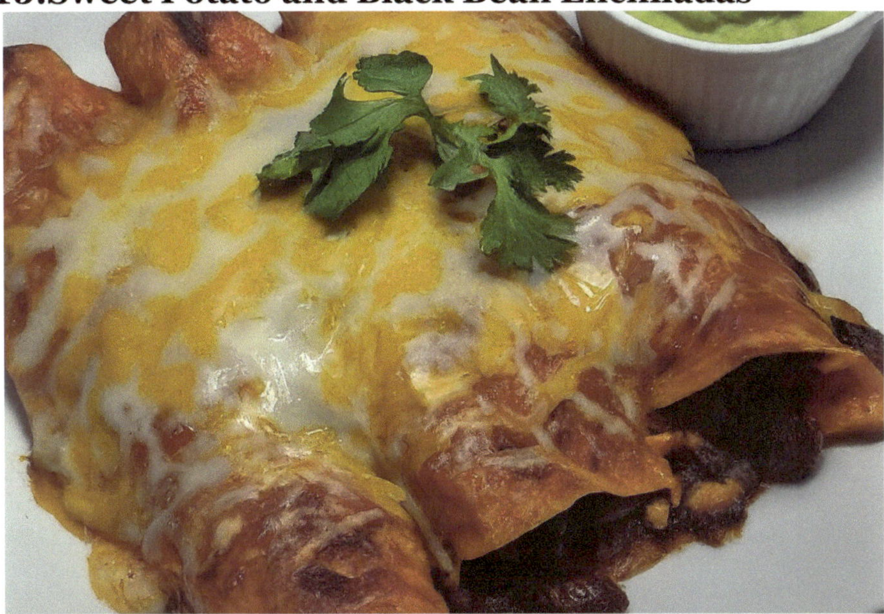

Ingredients

- 2 large sweet potatoes, peeled and diced
- 1 tablespoon olive oil
- 1 onion, diced
- 2 cloves garlic, minced
- 1 can (15 ounces) black beans, drained and rinsed
- 1 can (4 ounces) diced green chilies
- 1 teaspoon ground cumin
- 1/2 teaspoon chili powder
- Salt and pepper to taste
- 8 small whole wheat tortillas
- 2 cups enchilada sauce
- Vegan cheese, shredded (optional)
- Fresh cilantro, chopped (for garnish)
- Lime wedges (for serving)

Preparation

- Preheat the oven to 375°F (190°C).
- Place the diced sweet potatoes on a baking sheet and toss with olive oil. Roast in the preheated oven for about 25-30 minutes, or until tender.
- In a large pan, heat a small amount of olive oil over medium heat. Add the diced onion and minced garlic and sauté until softened.
- Add the black beans, diced green chilies, ground cumin, chili powder, salt, and pepper to the pan. Stir well to combine and cook for a few minutes.
- Warm the tortillas slightly to make them pliable.
- Pour a small amount of enchilada sauce into the bottom of a baking dish.
- Place a spoonful of the sweet potato and black bean mixture onto each tortilla, roll it up, and place it seam-side down in the baking dish.
- Once all the tortillas are filled and arranged in the baking dish, pour the remaining enchilada sauce over the top.
- If using, sprinkle the shredded vegan cheese over the enchiladas.
- Bake in the preheated oven for about 20-25 minutes, or until the enchiladas are heated through and the cheese is melted.
- Garnish with fresh cilantro and serve with lime wedges on the side.

Prep Time: 40 Minutes

Benefits:

Sweet potatoes provide fiber, vitamins, and minerals that cut cholesterol and inflammation. Black beans provide fiber and plant-based protein, which may decrease cholesterol and improve heart health. This vegetarian recipe is heart-healthy since it has minimal saturated fat and cholesterol. These heart-healthy Sweet Potato and Black Bean Enchiladas make a tasty vegetarian supper.

16. Kale Caesar Salad with Almond Croutons

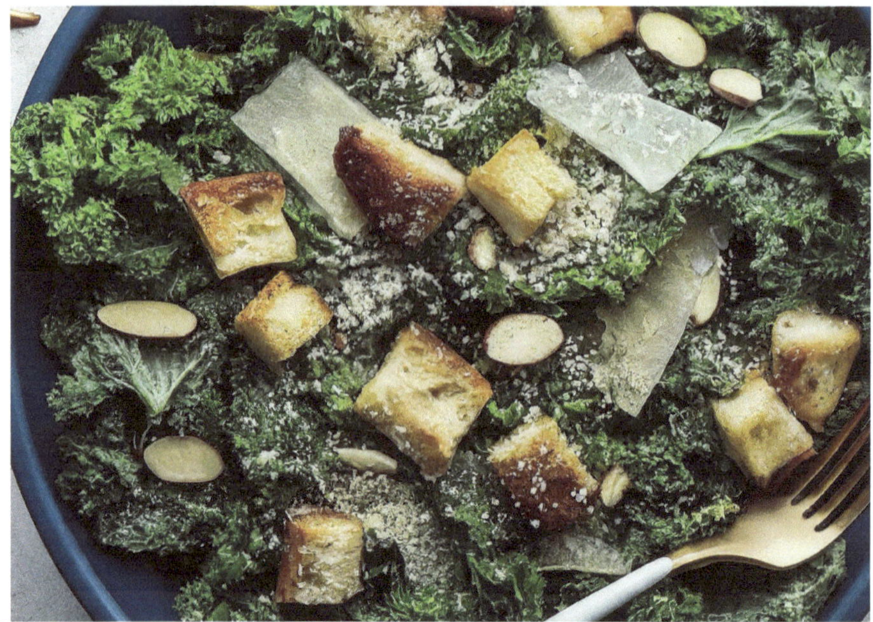

Ingredients

- 1 bunch of kale, stems removed and leaves torn into bite-sized pieces
- 1/4 cup almond slices
- 2 tablespoons olive oil
- 1 tablespoon lemon juice
- 1 clove garlic, minced
- 1 teaspoon Dijon mustard
- 1/4 cup grated Parmesan cheese
- Salt and pepper to taste
-

Prep Time:
30 Minutes

Preparation

- Preheat the oven to 350°F (175°C).
- Spread the almond slices on a baking sheet and toast in the preheated oven for about 5-7 minutes, or until golden brown. Set aside to cool.
- In a large bowl, whisk together the olive oil, lemon juice, minced garlic, Dijon mustard, and grated Parmesan cheese to make the dressing.
- Add the torn kale leaves to the bowl and toss to coat the leaves evenly with the dressing.
- Let the kale sit for about 10-15 minutes to allow the flavors to meld and the leaves to soften slightly.
- Just before serving, sprinkle the toasted almond slices over the salad.
- Season with salt and pepper to taste.

Benefits:
Kale is rich in antioxidants, vitamins, and minerals, which promote heart health. Almonds include monounsaturated lipids that may decrease cholesterol. A lighter, healthier Caesar salad, this salad is heart-healthy.

17. Asian Quinoa Salad Bowl

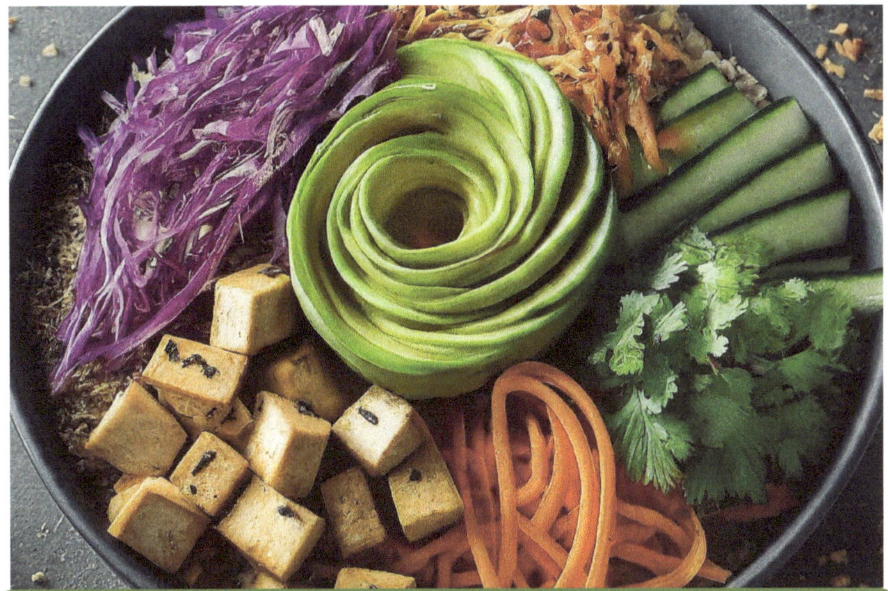

Ingredients

- 1 cup quinoa
- 2 cups water or vegetable broth
- 1 cup shredded red cabbage
- 1 cup shredded carrots
- 1 red bell pepper, thinly sliced
- 1/4 cup chopped cilantro
- 1/4 cup chopped green onions
- 1/4 cup roasted peanuts or cashews
- Sesame seeds (for garnish)
- For the Dressing:
- 3 tablespoons soy sauce
- 2 tablespoons rice vinegar
- 1 tablespoon sesame oil
- 1 tablespoon honey or maple syrup
- 1 teaspoon grated ginger
- 1 clove garlic, minced
- Red pepper flakes (optional, for heat)

Preparation

- Clean quinoa in cool water.
- Boil water or veggie broth in a pot. After adding the quinoa, decrease the heat to low, cover, and simmer for 15-20 minutes to cook and absorb the liquid. Fork-fluff and cool.
- Mix cooked quinoa, red cabbage, carrots, red bell pepper, cilantro, and green onions in a large bowl.
- Mix soy sauce, rice vinegar, sesame oil, honey or maple syrup, grated ginger, chopped garlic, and red pepper flakes (if used) in a small bowl to create the dressing.
- Toss the quinoa and vegetables with the dressing to coat.
- Serve the salad in dishes with roasted peanuts or cashews and sesame seeds.
- Benefits in Reversing Heart Diseases:
- Quinoa is a whole grain that is high in fiber and protein, which can help lower cholesterol levels and support heart health.
- The vegetables in this salad, such as red cabbage, carrots, and bell pepper, are rich in antioxidants and nutrients that may help reduce the risk of heart disease.
- Nuts like peanuts or cashews provide heart-healthy fats and may help lower the risk of heart disease.

Prep Time:
45 Minutes

Benefits:

Quinoa, a complete grain packed in fiber and protein, helps decrease cholesterol and promote heart health. Red cabbage, carrots, and bell pepper in this salad include antioxidants and minerals that may lower heart disease risk. Peanuts and cashews include heart-healthy lipids that may reduce heart disease risk.

20

18. Avocado and Mango Salad

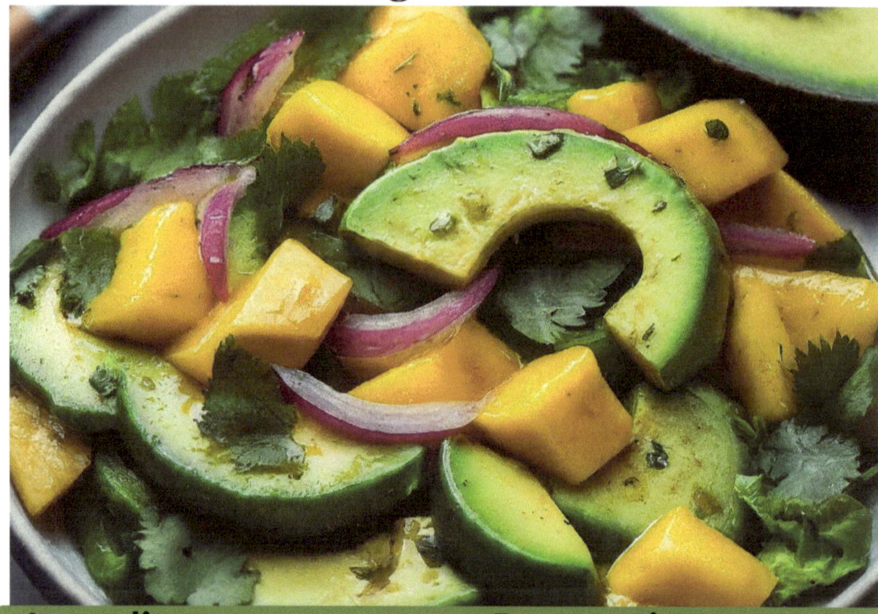

Ingredients

- 2 ripe avocados, peeled, pitted, and diced
- 2 ripe mangoes, peeled, pitted, and diced
- 1/4 cup red onion, finely chopped
- 1/4 cup fresh cilantro, chopped
- 1 jalapeño, seeded and finely chopped
- 2 tablespoons lime juice
- Salt and pepper to taste

Prep Time:
20 Minutes

Preparation

- In a large bowl, gently toss together the diced avocados, diced mangoes, chopped red onion, chopped cilantro, and chopped jalapeño.
- Drizzle the lime juice over the salad and gently toss to coat the ingredients.
- Season with salt and pepper to taste.
- Serve the avocado and mango salad immediately as a refreshing side dish or a light and flavorful appetizer.

Benefits:

Avocados provide vitamins and minerals and heart-healthy monounsaturated fats that may cut cholesterol and heart disease risk. Mangoes provide fiber, vitamins, and antioxidants that cut cholesterol and inflammation. A heart-healthy diet includes this vivid and nutritious salad.

19. Roasted Butternut Squash and Kale Salad

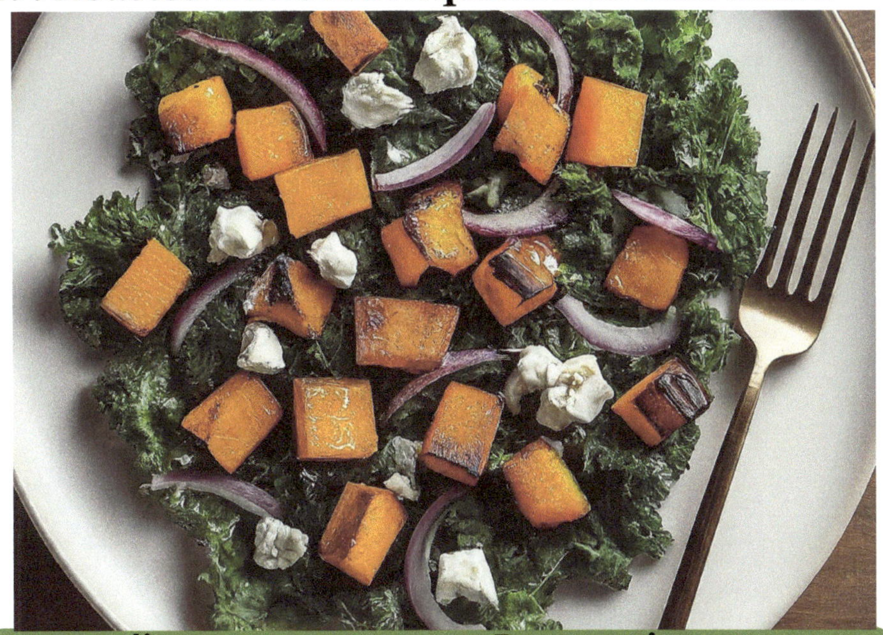

Ingredients

- 2 lb butternut squash, peeled, seeded, and cut into 1-inch cubes
- 1-2 tsp avocado oil or olive oil
- Salt and pepper to taste
- 4-5 cups chopped curly kale
- 15 oz canned chickpeas, drained and rinsed
- 1 cup fresh cranberries
- Honey for drizzling
- 1/2 cup crumbled feta cheese (optional)
- Crispy Chickpea Seasoning Blend:
- 1/2 tsp smoked paprika
- 1/2 tsp garlic powder
- 1/2 tsp ground cayenne pepper
- 1/2 tsp ground cumin
- 1/2 tsp black pepper
- Zesty Orange Dressing:
- 2 tbsp avocado oil or olive oil
- 2 tbsp orange juice
- 2 tsp apple cider vinegar
- 1/2 tsp salt
- 1/2 tsp pepper

Preparation

- Preheat oven to 400°F (200°C).
- Salt and pepper avocado or olive oil-coated butternut squash cubes. Spread them on a baking sheet and roast until tender and golden brown, 25–30 minutes.
- Mix avocado, kale, and collard greens in a big bowl.
- Mix the chickpeas and crispy chickpea seasoning in a separate bowl. Roast them on a baking sheet for 20–25 minutes until crisp.
- In a small saucepan, heat honey and cranberries over medium heat until they burst. Set aside.
- Mix the zesty orange dressing ingredients in a small bowl.
- After cooking, combine the butternut squash, chickpeas, and cranberries with massaged kale and collard greens.
- Pour spicy orange dressing over the salad and mix thoroughly.
- If using, crumble feta over salad.

**Prep Time:
30-45 Minutes**

Benefits:

Butternut squash has fiber, vitamins, and minerals that decrease cholesterol and inflammation.
Kale is rich in antioxidants, vitamins, and minerals, which promote heart health.
This salad adds taste and nutrition to a heart-healthy diet.

20. Carrot and Ginger Soup

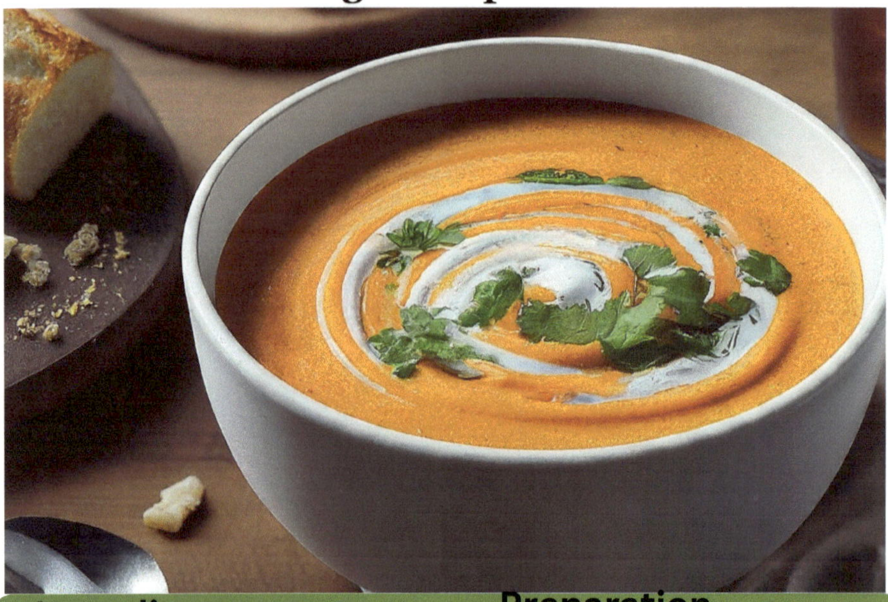

Ingredients

- 1 tablespoon olive oil
- 1 onion, chopped
- 2 cloves garlic, minced
- 1 tablespoon fresh ginger, grated
- 1 lb carrots, peeled and chopped
- 4 cups vegetable broth
- Salt and pepper to taste
- Fresh cilantro or parsley, for garnish

**Prep Time:
20-30 Minutes**

Preparation

- In a big saucepan, heat olive oil on medium. Add chopped onion and sauté until softened.
- Add minced garlic and grated ginger to the saucepan. Sauté another minute until fragrant.
- Put chopped carrots and vegetable broth in the saucepan. After boiling, lower heat to simmer. Cook carrots for 20–25 minutes until soft.
- Blend the soup using an immersion blender. You may also puree the soup in batches and return it to the saucepan.
- Salt and pepper the soup to taste. Garnish carrot and ginger soup with fresh cilantro or parsley and serve hot.

Benefits:

Beta-carotene, fiber, and antioxidants in carrots cut cholesterol and inflammation. Ginger has antioxidant and anti-inflammatory qualities that may aid the heart. This soup has minimal saturated fat and cholesterol, making it heart-healthy.

23

21. Spicy Tomato and Lentil Soup

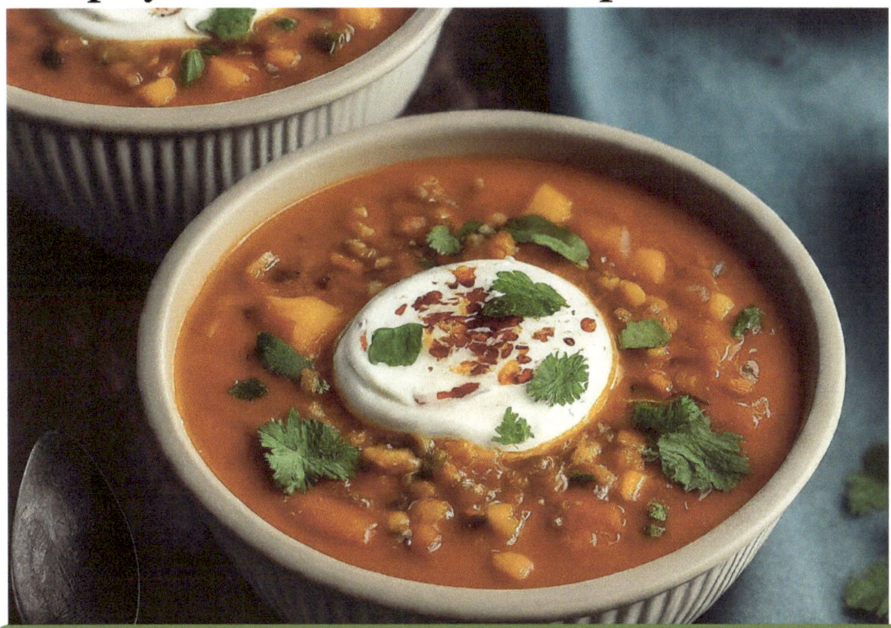

Ingredients

- 1 tablespoon olive oil
- 1 onion, diced
- 2 cloves garlic, minced
- 1 teaspoon ground cumin
- 1/2 teaspoon ground coriander
- 1/2 teaspoon smoked paprika
- 1/4 teaspoon cayenne pepper (adjust to taste)
- 1 cup dried red lentils, rinsed and drained
- 1 can (14 ounces) diced tomatoes
- 4 cups vegetable broth
- Salt and pepper to taste
- Fresh cilantro, for garnish

Preparation

- In a big saucepan, heat olive oil on medium. Add chopped onion and sauté until transparent.
- Mix minced garlic, ground cumin, coriander, smoked paprika, and cayenne pepper in the saucepan. Cook until aromatic, 1-2 minutes.
- Put washed red lentils, diced tomatoes, and vegetable broth in the saucepan. After boiling, lower heat to simmer. Cook lentils for 20–25 minutes until cooked.
- Salt and pepper the soup to taste.
- Add fresh cilantro to the spicy tomato and lentil soup and serve hot.

**Prep Time:
10 Minutes**

Benefits:

Lentils are abundant in fiber and protein, which decrease cholesterol and improve heart health. Lycopene, an antioxidant, is abundant in tomatoes and may lower heart disease risk. This soup is heart-healthy since it has minimal saturated fat and cholesterol.

22. Moroccan Chickpea Stew

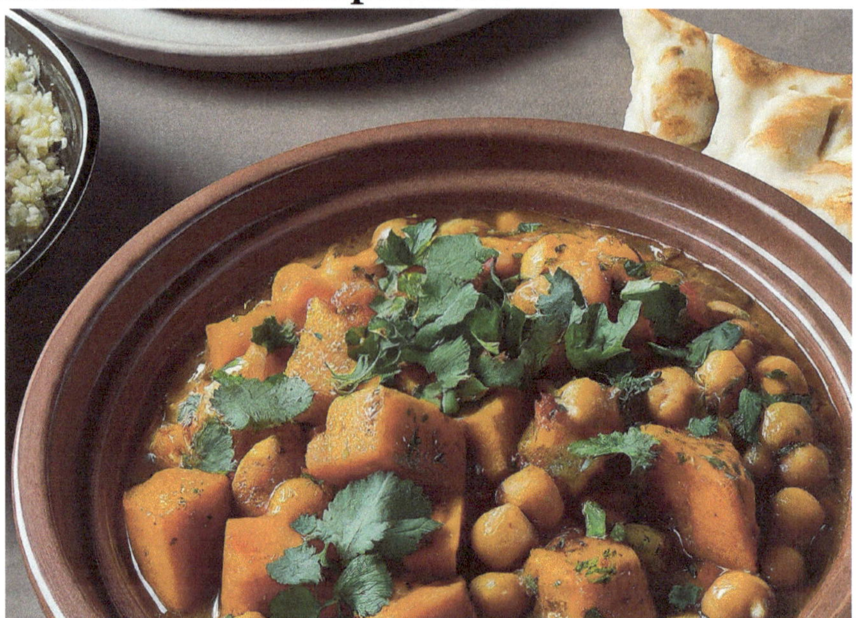

Ingredients

- 2 tablespoons olive oil
- 1 onion, diced
- 3 cloves garlic, minced
- 1 teaspoon ground cumin
- 1/2 teaspoon ground turmeric
- 1/2 teaspoon ground cinnamon
- 1/2 teaspoon ground ginger
- 1 can (15-ounce) crushed tomatoes
- 1 tablespoon harissa paste
- 8 cups vegetable stock or water
- 1 cup fresh cilantro, chopped, divided
- 1 cup lentils
- 1 can (15-ounce) chickpeas, drained
- Salt to taste
- Lemon wedges, for serving
- Greek yogurt and toasted almonds for topping (optional)

Preparation

- Preheat your oven to 400°F (200°C).
- On a bakHeat the olive oil in a large pot over medium heat. Add the diced onion and cook until softened, about 5 minutes.
- Add the minced garlic, ground cumin, ground turmeric, ground cinnamon, and ground ginger to the pot. Cook for about 1-2 minutes until fragrant.
- Stir in the crushed tomatoes and harissa paste. Cook for another 2 minutes, allowing the flavors to meld together.
- Add the vegetable stock or water and half of the chopped cilantro to the pot. Stir well to combine.
- Add the lentils and drained chickpeas to the pot. Bring the stew to a boil, then reduce the heat and simmer for about 30-35 minutes, or until the lentils are tender.
- Season the stew with salt to taste.
- Serve the Moroccan chickpea stew hot, garnished with the remaining fresh cilantro. Squeeze fresh lemon juice over each serving. You can also top the stew with a dollop of Greek yogurt and toasted almonds for added flavor and texture.
- ing sheet, combine the Brussels sprouts and beets with olive oil, salt, and pepper.
- Roast in a preheated oven for 20-25 minutes, or until the veggies are soft and faintly caramelized.
- In a serving bowl, mix together the roasted Brussels sprouts and beets.
- Sprinkle with toasted walnuts and crumbled goat cheese.
- Drizzle with honey-Dijon vinaigrette before serving.

Prep Time:
30 Minutes

Benefits:

Lentils provide fiber and protein, which cut cholesterol and heart disease risk. Chickpeas are rich in fiber and contain heart-healthy nutrients like folate and magnesium. The spices used in this stew, such as cumin, turmeric, cinnamon, and ginger, have anti-inflammatory properties and may help support heart health. This stew is low in saturated fat and cholesterol, making it a heart-healthy option.

25

23. Creamy Mushroom and Wild Rice Soup

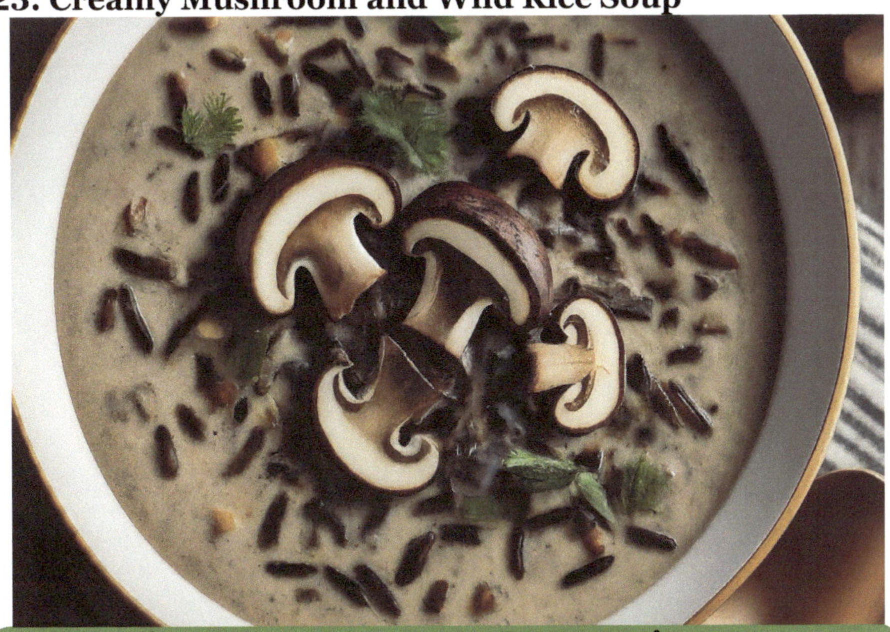

Ingredients

- 2 tablespoons olive oil
- 1 onion, diced
- 3 cloves garlic, minced
- 8 ounces mushrooms, sliced
- 1/4 cup all-purpose flour
- 4 cups vegetable broth
- 1 cup unsweetened almond milk (or any non-dairy milk)
- 1 cup cooked wild rice
- 1 teaspoon dried thyme
- Salt and pepper to taste
- Fresh parsley, for garnish

Preparation

- Heat olive oil in a big saucepan on medium. Cook the chopped onion for 5 minutes to soften.
- Insert minced garlic and mushroom slices into the pot. Cook mushrooms for 8-10 minutes until they release moisture and brown.
- Sprinkle all-purpose flour over mushrooms and mix thoroughly. Cook for 2 more minutes to eliminate raw flour flavor.
- To avoid lumps, slowly add vegetable broth while stirring. Simmer the soup.
- Almond milk, cooked wild rice, dried thyme, salt, and pepper should be added to the saucepan on low heat. Mix thoroughly.
- Simmer the soup for 20–25 minutes to blend flavors and thicken.
- Season with salt and pepper as required.
- Top the creamy mushroom and wild rice soup with fresh parsley and serve hot.

Prep Time:

1 Hr

Benefits:

Some of the chemicals found in mushrooms have the potential to decrease cholesterol and lessen the likelihood of cardiovascular disease. A nutrient-dense grain, wild rice is rich in fiber and has the potential to reduce cholesterol. This soup is great for your heart since it's low in cholesterol and saturated fat.

24. Butternut Squash and Apple Soup

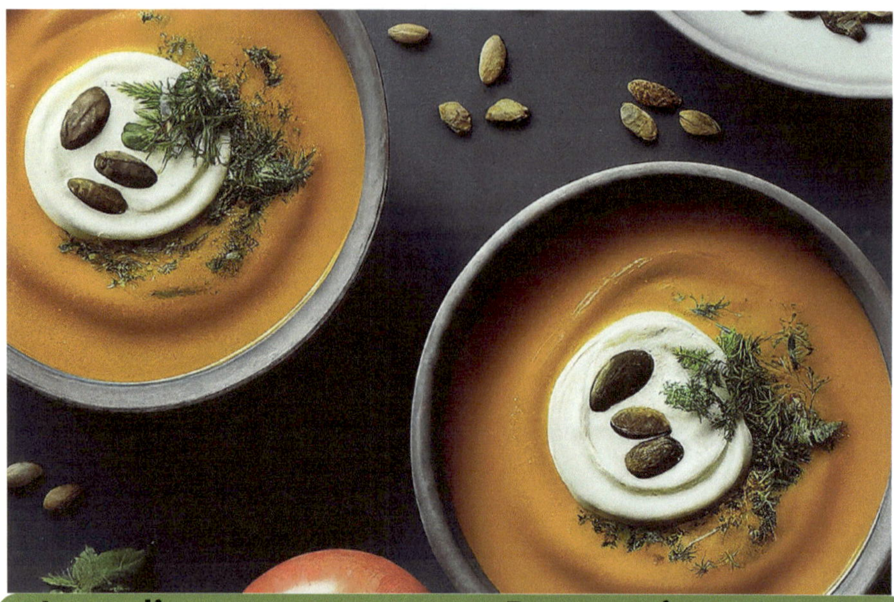

Ingredients

- 1 butternut squash, peeled, seeded, and cubed
- 2 apples, peeled, cored, and chopped
- 1 onion, chopped
- 3 cloves garlic, minced
- 4 cups vegetable broth
- 1 teaspoon ground cinnamon
- 1/2 teaspoon ground nutmeg
- Salt and pepper to taste
- Olive oil for drizzling
- Pumpkin seeds, for garnish

Prep Time:
25 Minutes

Preparation

- Turn the oven on high heat (400°F, 200°C).
- Prepare a baking sheet by arranging the cubes of butternut squash, chopped apples, diced onion, and minced garlic. Add the olive oil and mix to combine.
- To produce soft and caramelized veggies and apples, roast them in a preheated oven for 30–35 minutes.
- In a big saucepan, add the roasted apples and veggies. Season with pepper, cinnamon, nutmeg, salt, and vegetable broth.
- Reduce the heat to low when the mixture has boiled. Put it on low heat for ten to fifteen minutes so the flavors can combine.
- Smooth out the soup by pureeing it with an immersion blender. Another option is to split the soup into smaller portions and puree them in a blender until they are smooth. Then, add them back to the saucepan.
- Add more salt and pepper to taste to the soup.
- Hot soup made with butternut squash and apples is best served with pumpkin seeds sprinkled on top.

Benefits:

A decreased blood pressure and reduced risk of heart disease may be possible benefits of eating butternut squash due to its high potassium, fiber, and vitamin A and C content. In addition to lowering cholesterol and inflammation, the high quantities of dietary fiber and antioxidants found in apples make them a heart-healthy food choice. This soup is great for your heart since it's low in cholesterol and saturated fat.

25. Pumpkin and Black Bean Casserole

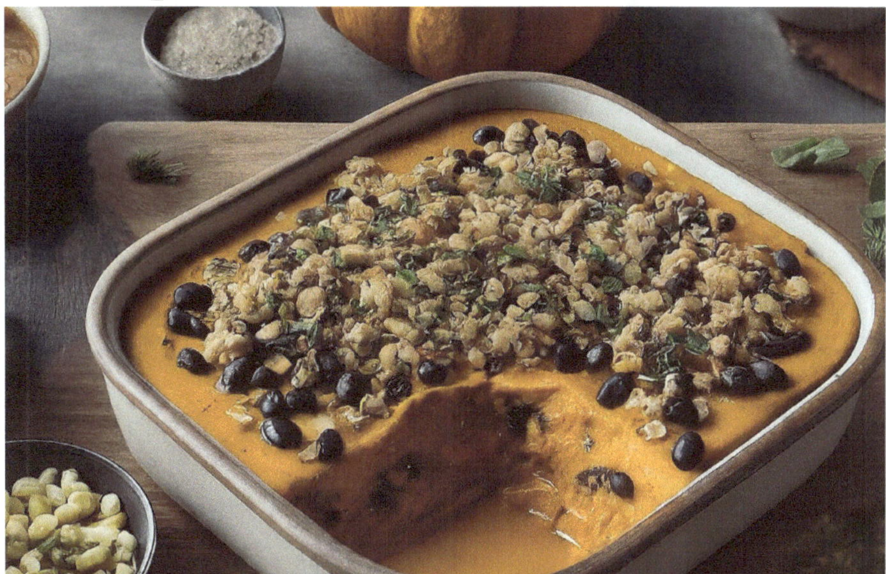

Ingredients

- 2 cups cooked black beans
- 2 cups pumpkin puree
- 1 onion, diced
- 2 cloves garlic, minced
- 1 red bell pepper, diced
- 1 green bell pepper, diced
- 1 cup corn kernels
- 1 can (14 ounces) diced tomatoes
- 1 teaspoon ground cumin
- 1 teaspoon chili powder
- Salt and pepper to taste
- 1 cup shredded vegan cheese (optional)
- Fresh cilantro, for garnish

**Prep Time:
1 hr 15 Minutes**

Preparation

- A preheated oven of 375 degrees Fahrenheit (190 degrees Celsius) is required.
- Cook the bell peppers, onion, and garlic in a big pan over medium heat until they are softened.
- Spice up your pan with a combination of cooked black beans, pumpkin puree, corn kernels, chopped tomatoes (together with their juice), ground cumin, chili powder, salt, and pepper. Coat well to blend.
- To make sure all the flavors combine, cook the mixture for around five to seven minutes. Taste and add more spice as required.
- Spread the mixture evenly in a casserole dish after transferring it.
- Shredded vegan cheese may be sprinkled on top of the dish if preferred.
- The dish should be warm and bubbling after 30–35 minutes in a preheated oven.
- Serve with a sprinkle of fresh cilantro as a garnish.

Benefits:

The heart-healthy minerals magnesium and folate found in black beans complement their high fiber content. Pumpkin may help decrease blood pressure and lessen the risk of heart disease because to its high potassium, fiber, and antioxidant content. Because it contains less cholesterol and saturated fat, this dish is good for your heart.

26. Vegan Jambalaya with Jackfruit

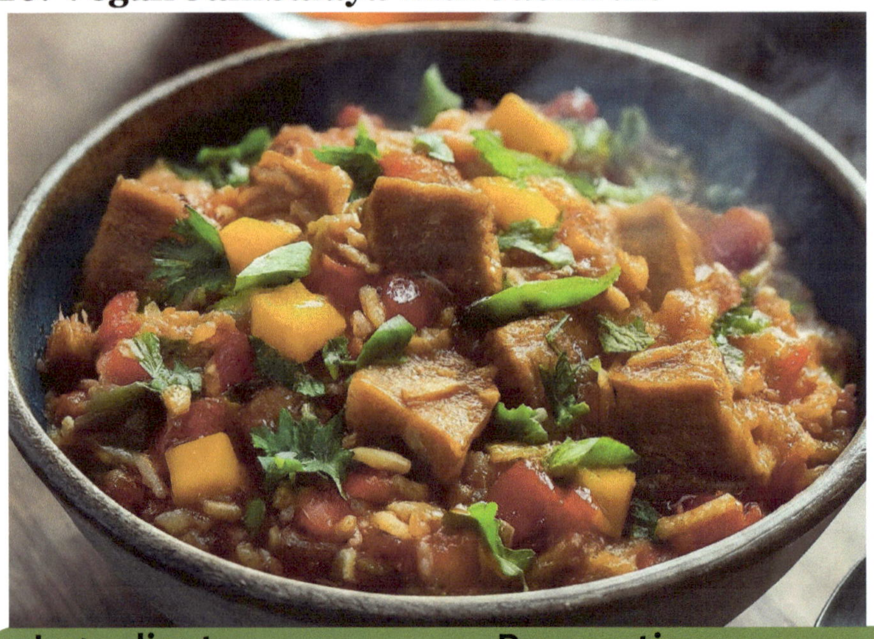

Ingredients

- 2 tablespoons olive oil
- 1 onion, diced
- 3 cloves garlic, minced
- 1 green bell pepper, diced
- 1 red bell pepper, diced
- 2 celery stalks, diced
- 1 can (14 ounces) diced tomatoes
- 1 can (14 ounces) young jackfruit, drained and rinsed
- 1 cup long-grain brown rice
- 2 cups vegetable broth
- 1 tablespoon Cajun seasoning
- 1 teaspoon dried thyme
- 1 teaspoon smoked paprika
- Salt and pepper to taste
- Fresh parsley, for garnish

Prep Time:
1hr 15 Minutes

Preparation

- Heat the olive oil in a large pot over medium heat. Add the diced onion, minced garlic, diced bell peppers, and diced celery. Sauté until the vegetables are softened.
- Add the diced tomatoes, young jackfruit, brown rice, vegetable broth, Cajun seasoning, dried thyme, smoked paprika, salt, and pepper to the pot. Stir well to combine.
- Bring the mixture to a boil, then reduce the heat to low. Cover the pot and simmer for about 45-50 minutes, or until the rice is cooked and the flavors have melded together.
- Adjust the seasoning with salt and pepper if needed.
- Serve the vegan jambalaya hot, garnished with fresh parsley.

Benefits:

Jackfruit, a multipurpose fruit, may stand in for meat when it comes to plant-based diets. Because of its low cholesterol and saturated fat content, it is a good choice for heart health. A complete grain, brown rice has a lot of fiber and may help reduce cholesterol. Thanks to its abundance of veggies and lack of meat, this jambalaya is a great choice for those watching their cholesterol levels and heart health.

29

27. Spaghetti Squash with Pesto and Cherry Tomatoes

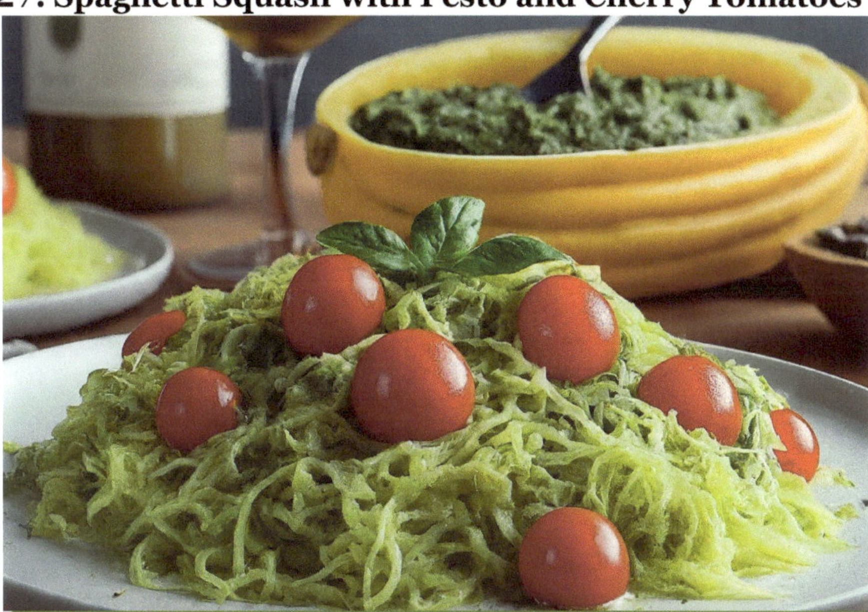

Ingredients

- 1 spaghetti squash
- 1 cup fresh basil leaves
- 1/4 cup pine nuts
- 2 cloves garlic
- 1/4 cup extra-virgin olive oil
- 2 tablespoons nutritional yeast
- Salt and pepper to taste
- Cherry tomatoes, halved, for garnish
- Fresh basil leaves, for garnish

Prep Time: 60 Min.

Preparation

1. Preheat the oven to 400°F (200°C).
2. Cut the spaghetti squash in half lengthwise and scoop out the seeds.
3. Place the squash halves cut-side down on a baking sheet. Roast in the preheated oven for about 40-45 minutes, or until the squash is tender and the strands can be easily scraped out with a fork.
4. While the squash is roasting, prepare the pesto. In a food processor, combine the fresh basil leaves, pine nuts, garlic, extra-virgin olive oil, nutritional yeast, salt, and pepper. Process until the ingredients are well combined and form a smooth pesto sauce.
5. Once the squash is cooked, remove it from the oven and let it cool slightly. Use a fork to scrape the strands of the squash into a bowl, separating them to resemble spaghetti.
6. Add the pesto sauce to the spaghetti squash strands and toss well to coat.
7. Serve the spaghetti squash with pesto and cherry tomatoes. Garnish with fresh basil leaves.
8.

Benefits:

Spaghetti squash is a low-calorie and low-carbohydrate alternative to traditional pasta, making it a heart-healthy option for those watching their weight and blood sugar levels. Basil is rich in antioxidants and has anti-inflammatory properties that may benefit heart health. This dish is free from refined grains and added sugars, making it a heart-healthy and diabetes-friendly option.

30

28. Grilled Salmon with Lemon and Dill

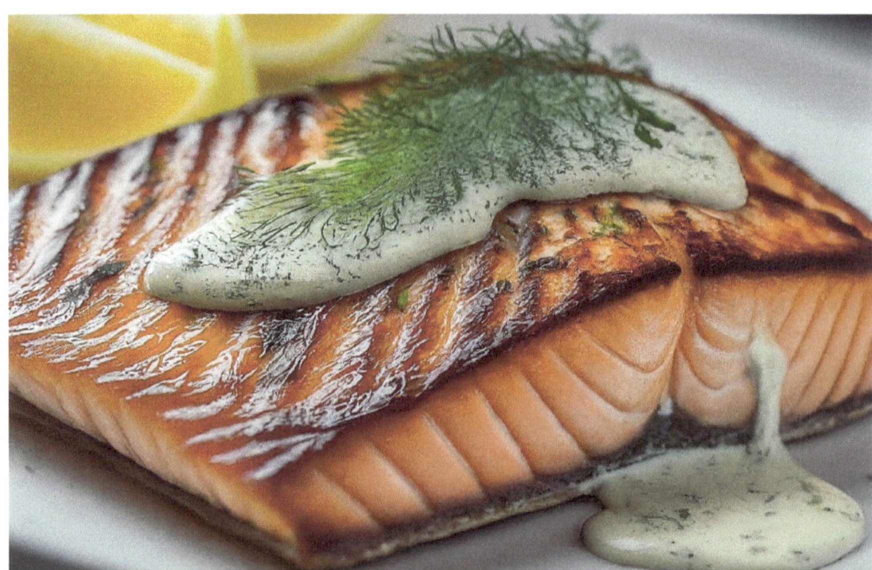

Ingredients

- 4 salmon fillets
- 2 tablespoons olive oil
- 2 cloves garlic, minced
- 2 tablespoons fresh dill, chopped
- 1 lemon, sliced
- Salt and pepper to taste

Prep Time: 20 Minutes

Preparation

- Turn the grill on high heat and let it heat up.
- The olive oil, garlic, and dill should be combined in a small bowl.
- Before brushing the salmon fillets with the olive oil mixture, season them with salt and pepper.
- To keep the salmon fillets from adhering to the grill, lay the lemon slices on top.
- To make the salmon opaque and flaky, grill it for four to five minutes each side.
- Garnish the grilled salmon with a dash of fresh dill and extra slices of lemon.

Benefits:

Salmon is a rich source of omega-3 fatty acids, which are known to reduce the risk of heart disease. Omega-3 fatty acids can help lower blood pressure, reduce the risk of blood clots, and decrease inflammation in the body, all of which contribute to heart health.

31

29. Baked Chicken Breast with Herbs

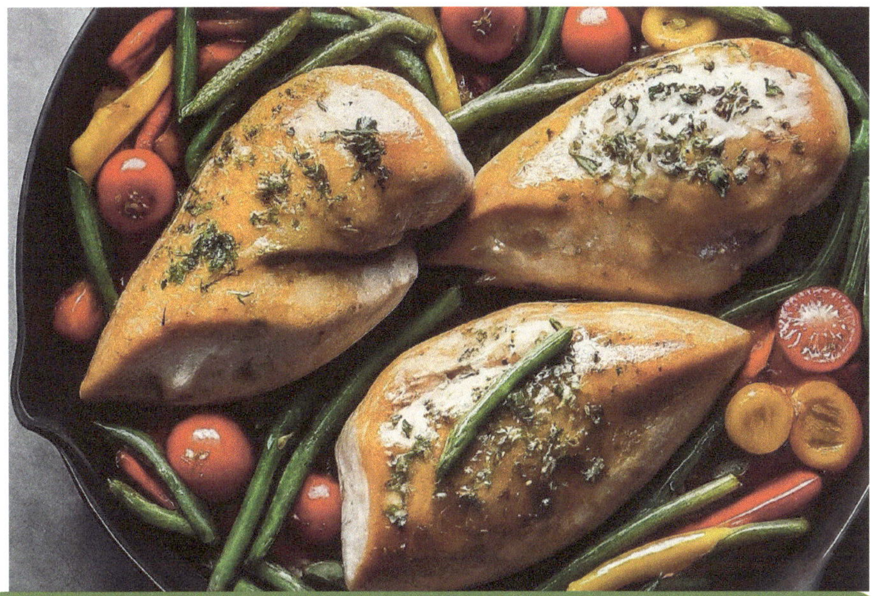

Ingredients

- 4 boneless, skinless chicken breasts
- 2 tablespoons olive oil
- 2 cloves garlic, minced
- 1 teaspoon dried rosemary
- 1 teaspoon dried thyme
- 1 teaspoon dried oregano
- Salt and pepper to taste
- Fresh parsley, for garnish

Prep Time: 40 Minutes

Preparation

- Set the oven temperature to 400°F, or 200°C.
- Second, in a baking dish, lay the chicken breasts. Add olive oil, then season with salt, pepper, dried rosemary, thyme, oregano, and chopped garlic.
- 3. Coat the chicken evenly with the spices by rubbing it in with your hands.
- 4. After the oven is warm, bake the chicken for 25 to 30 minutes, or until it reaches an internal temperature of 165 degrees Fahrenheit (74 degrees Celsius).
- Serve with a sprinkle of fresh parsley for garnish.

Benefits:

When compared to red meat, chicken has less saturated fat and is a leaner protein source. Incorporating lean proteins into a well-rounded diet may support heart health by assisting with weight maintenance and lowering the risk of cardiovascular disease.

30. Turkey and Vegetable Stir-Fry

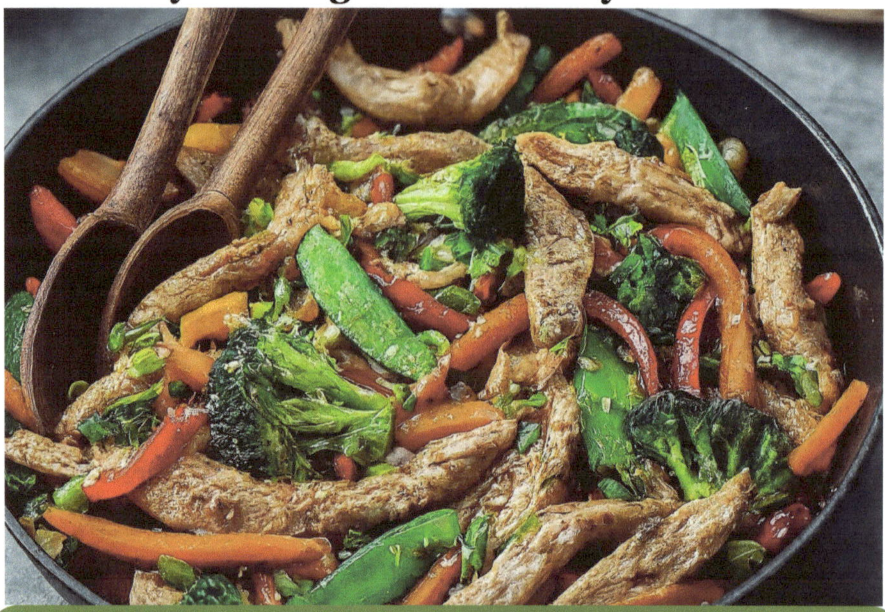

Ingredients

- 1 lb (450g) ground turkey
- 2 tablespoons olive oil
- 2 cloves garlic, minced
- 1-inch piece of ginger, grated
- 1 red bell pepper, thinly sliced
- 1 yellow bell pepper, thinly sliced
- 1 small zucchini, thinly sliced
- 1 cup snap peas
- 2 tablespoons low-sodium soy sauce
- 1 tablespoon honey or maple syrup
- 1 tablespoon cornstarch
- 1/4 cup water
- Salt and pepper to taste
- Sesame seeds, for garnish (optional)

Preparation

1. In a big pan or wok, heat the olive oil over medium-high heat.
2. Next, add the ground turkey and heat, stirring occasionally, until it becomes browned and fully cooked.
3. Cook for one more minute, or until aromatic, then add the grated ginger and minced garlic to the pan.
4. Toss in the pan with the cut zucchini, bell peppers, and snap peas. Cook, stirring occasionally, for three to four minutes, or until veggies are soft but still crunchy.
5. Combine the cornstarch, water, honey (or maple syrup), and soy sauce in a small bowl and whisk to combine.
6. After browning the turkey and veggies, pour sauce over them. To ensure a uniform coating, stir well.
7. To thicken the sauce, cook for an additional one to two minutes.
8. Add pepper and salt to taste.
9. Heat up some brown rice or quinoa and top it with the turkey and veggie stir-fry.
10. Sesame seeds may be used as a garnish if preferred.

Prep Time:
25 Minutes

Benefits:

As a lean protein source, ground turkey may aid with weight maintenance and lower the risk of cardiovascular disease. The veggies in this stir-fry are great for your heart since they are full of nutrients, fiber, and antioxidants. When compared to stir-fry sauces with a lot of salt, this one is better for your heart because of the low-sodium soy sauce and the few additional sweets..

Final Thougts

Delicious and healthy supper dishes with an emphasis on plant-based foods are yours to enjoy in this cookbook. Not only do we hope these dishes have been delicious, but we also hope they have motivated you to make long-term improvements to your diet.

Keep in mind that switching to a plant-based diet is an ongoing commitment to better health, not a quick cure. More fruits, veggies, whole grains, and legumes should be a regular part of your diet, and we hope you'll keep trying new plant-based recipes.

The "Reversing Heart Disease Cookbook" is an excellent choice to accompany you on your life-altering quest. Not only have these meals provided nourishment for your body, but we hope they have also given happiness and contentment to your dinner table.